How I Cured My Heartburn and Hiatal Hernia

By
Al Praktik

**Atlantach
Publishing**

An Atlantach Publication 2023
Cover design by M Gallagher at Le Chéile, Galway

Introduction

It's hard to even explain what heartburn feels like. Most of my relations on both sides of my family suffered with heartburn. Everyone seems to have a different description of what it is and what it feels like.

Lots of people say it's GERD, acid-reflux or simply indigestion, but the people who are suffering from it are in a horrible kind of misery. I have seen the same look of misery on the faces of many of my relatives.

When you are young you think they just have a tummy-ache, nothing more than a mere discomfort, nothing a few antacids can't take care of. Some of your relatives have different cures, baking soda and water, milk, antacids, PPI's, H2 blockers and more.

I can only describe heartburn as being a horrible burning sensation in my chest. I found the anticipation of getting heartburn just as miserable as the actual suffering of it.

I spent ten years suffering with heartburn and trying out all the 'cures' before I was finally called for a gastroscopy and diagnosed as having a hiatal hernia. A hiatal hernia occurs when the upper part of your stomach bulges through your diaphragm.

Chapter 1

What Causes Heartburn?

My maternal grandmother suffered terribly with heartburn until she had her gall-bladder removed - quite an operation in the 50's. My mother also suffered badly with heartburn until she had her gall-bladder removed in the 80's, and she is still on a PPI.

My half-brother suffered terribly with heartburn for many years before his untimely death from a heart-attack at the young age of 46. He suffered with hernias but I am not sure what kind of hernias they were.

These are just a few of the many members of my family that suffered with heartburn. My mother noticed a correlation between heartburn and heart trouble many years ago. My belief is that suffering with heartburn causes tremendous stress which eventually troubles the heart.

I have noticed that almost all of my male relatives who suffered with heartburn smoked heavily and this was labelled as the cause for their heartburn, alcohol was blamed also. Apparently, many women suffer bad heartburn while pregnant.

Many people have identified a certain food as being the cause of their heartburn and by avoiding that particular food they are able to manage their heartburn. I was suffering to the stage where I was getting heartburn no matter what I ate, but certainly, some foods were really strong 'triggers'.

I remember a packet of crisps/potato chips causing me such misery that I did not touch them again for over ten years.

One morning I ate two jambons on my way to work and I felt like I was having a heart-attack the whole day.

I could not drink much water because even that gave me heartburn. I preferred instead to drink milk or cola. I found somehow that the bubbles in cola seemed to help. Later on, I noticed that sparkling water helped also. Alcohol was a complete no-no.

My half-brother could not eat white bread unless it was toasted. In time, I too had the same problem.

White-pudding was another food I could not eat. Other foods I have heard people mention and some which I found troublesome are; tomatoes, stuffing, fry-ups, onions, garlic, rhubarb, breaded-fish, herbs, spices and many more.

It seems to me that if some foods you have been eating all of your life suddenly start giving you heartburn, then something else is 'causing' your heartburn.

Chapter 2

The Beginning

When I was in my early 30's I was working with a builder who was not much older than me and I noticed that he drank a lot of milk. The boss used to laugh at him, "You're like a suck-calf with all that milk you're drinking". He was drinking three to four 2liter bottles of milk every day at work. I asked him why he drank so much milk and he told me that it was the only thing that relieved his heartburn.

He was the first really serious case of heartburn that I took notice of. I mentioned my family members earlier but it was not until I had cured my own heartburn that I did a study of my family's heartburn, and by study, I mean just talking about it and what I remember. Up to this point I was in the pink of health and I remember being puzzled by his heartburn as he was relatively young, didn't smoke, was not terribly overweight and didn't drink that much alcohol. He went out at the weekends like we all did.

Up to this point I had never suffered with heartburn in my life so I could only imagine the pain he was going through, in fact I imagined it was nothing more than a discomfort when he was working away like everyone else.

It was some years later before I started to get heartburn. I had it a few times before I actually realized what it was and was able to describe it. I was not alarmed but I can remember being disappointed thinking that I was too young to be getting heartburn. I did not think to document the progression of my heartburn as I didn't think it was a serious problem, a few antacids used to relieve it.

As time went on, I remembered to keep a packet of antacids on my person when I was going for a few drinks. Pretty soon I had to make sure I had antacids any time I went for a fry-up. I can't remember exactly but within a year or two I seemed to be suffering a lot with heartburn. It was not long before I too was bringing 2liter bottles of milk into work.

Chapter 3

Alcohol

I can remember being in a pub one night and there was a darts trophy with brandy in it being passed around. Everybody was taking a sip to take part in the celebrations. I didn't like spirits but I took a small sip to join in and almost immediately, with that sip, I got the most painful, burning sensation in my chest. I felt really bad and I knew then there was something seriously wrong with me.

Of course, I made sure I never touched anything containing brandy or whiskey ever again.

Slowly and slowly there seemed to be more things to avoid but I hated brandy so that wasn't too bad. I could do without the white-pudding at breakfast time. No harm to cut out crisps, they are fattening. This is how I dealt with it as I had no choice, life goes on and you have to keep going. I can't remember exactly how long I was tolerating living like this but it was some years.

Even drinking beer was not worth the heartburn at nights and all day the next day so that was cut out as well in the hope I would get better.

Work was becoming more and more difficult. I read somewhere online that bending over repeatedly was not good for heartburn but I am a bricklayer so there was not much I could do about that only make sure I had three or four 2liter bottles of milk lying around.

Chapter 4

PPI's

Some years after first working with him, I met the builder who was drinking all the milk. He looked very well and I asked him if he still suffered with heartburn. He told me he had no problem at all anymore since he was prescribed to a PPI. This was my first-time hearing about them.

I was thrilled, not just for him but for me. Now I could go on this miraculous PPI. At long last, a cure. I was so happy. I called my doctor the very next day and a prescription was written out. Within a very short space of time, I had no heartburn. Oh God, what a relief to get rid of that horrible, miserable pain and the nerves associated with the anticipation of the onset of heartburn. In my view, the stress caused by the anticipation of heartburn is just as bad as the heartburn itself. Every time I ate or drank anything I was wondering was I going to be tortured by heartburn.

After a little while on the PPI I started to feel great, naturally when your pain and misery is taken away that is how you will feel. I felt so good that I wanted to go back boxing again. I had a very disappointing professional boxing career resulting in my retirement at a relatively young age. Now with my heartburn gone I felt like a new man.

Chapter 5

Vaping

As I have stated, I never kept a detailed timeline of the sickness from my heartburn as I did not think it was going to be such a debilitating condition as it turned out to be. I know for certain that it was at the very least ten years I suffered from it because my half-brother died at 46 and I was definitely afflicted with it at that time and I was 36. I cured it when I was 46, just in the nick of time I believe.

Although I do not have any proof, I believe that vaping caused me a lot of damage internally. I say this purely from a layman's point of view, I believe the nicotine I was inhaling did the damage to me. The hiatal hernia was located right at the base of my lungs. I believe the nicotine 'settled' there and did the damage.

I took up vaping as a 'healthy' alternative to smoking. At that time, it was believed that the tar in cigarettes was the big problem. A few of my friends were very happy with the transition from smoking to vaping and highly recommended it to me.

I absolutely loved my roll-ups during brief periods of retirement from boxing and I always claimed that I would take up a 'healthy' smoking habit should a healthy alternative be provided - well here it was and I embraced it. I thought it was just fantastic. You could vape everywhere and anywhere and that I did, practically every minute of the day. At least a roll-up will go out eventually and you will have to spend a little time rolling another one, but once you have a spare battery cigarette, the vaping need never stop.

I did not eat nearly as much while I was vaping and as a consequence, I lost a few pounds and actually looked a bit 'ripped' but I was not healthy and vaping was just half of the problem.

Chapter 6

Sore Elbow

Although my boxing training was going quite well, I was concerned that my face had turned quite a bright red. I was rather alarmed and subject to ridicule. Again, disappointed, I just assumed it was a part of aging. My half-brother's face was also quite red when he was the same age. Actually, I knew quite a few people with red faces so it was quite normal if a bit embarrassing. At least with the embarrassment I had a reason to have a red face.

My new-found elation from ridding myself of heartburn was soon replaced with a dull, throbbing, constantly painful elbow. Honestly, it is hard to say which was worse, the heartburn or the elbow. I tried every pain-relief known to man to no avail. My boxing training obviously was not going well with this condition and strength-training basically had to stop, it was too painful and I was too tired.

The elbow was sapping the very life out of me. It made my work life extremely difficult. A lot of weight goes through a bricklayer's elbow every day. I started to decline work on Saturdays in an effort to rest my elbow in an attempt to be fresh on Mondays. Right away, this put a strain on me financially.

You might think that "It's just one day" but if you live in London, as I was at the time, that one day might double your disposable income. I mean, after you have paid your rent and bills, you might only have a day or two of disposable income left.

Luckily, I didn't drink so I didn't need a lot of money to get by. As time went on, I started missing days during the week at times when things weren't too busy. This was sheer tiredness from the sapping pain of the elbow. I noticed my body weakening rapidly and healing-time was very slow in the event of injuries.

Chapter 7

Giving up Vaping

I tried many times to give up vaping but I was unable to. I decided to go back smoking roll-ups to replace the vaping. After a couple of months, I was able to give up smoking again. Almost immediately after giving up vaping my elbow improved a little but it has never fully recovered.

After many hours a week on the internet looking for cures for sore elbows, I learned a few tips from other bricklayers on some internet forums. The best tip by far was to use a smaller trowel. You might think this is obvious but I didn't know about it or think it would make much difference. It made a vast difference.

Another tip was not to bed out too far in front of you. 'Bedding out' is quite simply laying the mortar on the bricks in preparation for another brick to be laid on top of it. Bedding out is tiring on the elbow so it is better to use just one trowel-full of mortar and lay your brick or two, then bed out one trowel-full again. This breaks up the movement a bit and takes a little strain of the elbow.

A final bit of advice I learned on some forum was also valuable. A bricklayer mentioned that he had this habit of constantly 'knocking-up' (mixing) his mortar on the spot boards to keep it at an optimal freshness. I noticed that I had the same habit. He said to just keep using the fresh stuff at the top and before long you won't have a very large amount of muck left on the spot board to knock-up which will save your elbow a lot of work. Of course, he was right, it was just a bad habit.

At least through a few small changes I was able to get back to work a bit better and do a decent day's work again.

Chapter 8

H Pylori

I met a few people who gave up smoking and took up vaping in an effort to live a healthier life. A couple of them developed a sore elbow. I have also met a couple of people who got a sore elbow while just on PPI's alone, so I am not sure what is worse but I suspect that both of them together are very bad. A quick investigation into PPI's will tell you that they work by cutting down your stomach acid. Cut down your stomach acid and you are not digesting your food optimally and you are going to miss out on valuable minerals and nutrients. When this happens, you start getting ailments and healing time slows. It's all related.

Just when I thought things couldn't get worse, I started developing chronic back pain. Life was really miserable at this stage. I felt like a really old man and time was marching on. I was 41 by now and I never got fit enough to make a return to the ring and I packed in the boxing.

With more spare time on my hands, I spent more time on the computer trying to find out what was wrong with me and see if I could cure myself.

There seems to be very little information on the internet about heartburn. There's lots and lots of content but no real information.

The same can be said about a sore-elbow. You will see it classified as tendonitis, golfer's elbow and tennis elbow, again, lots and lots of content but no real information.

One thing I learned on the internet was to incline my bed. I found this helped a little to prevent heartburn at night and it helped my sore back. I also slept a little better.

I tried lots of different things to cure heartburn and I was fast approaching the age at which my half-brother died and this did not help with stress.

My doctor put me on a course of antibiotics in case I had a h pylori infection. The moment I discontinued my PPI's I got the worst heartburn so I quickly went back on them. I wanted to get off PPI's but I didn't want to be suffering with heartburn.

Chapter 9

Ditching the PPI's

By now I had a bad back, sore elbow, low energy, little strength and didn't feel well generally but as long as I was on my PPI I was not suffering with heartburn.

Now my weight was getting to be a concern. Naturally I expected to put on a little weight as I was getting older and had finished boxing but I knew intuitively that there were other factors at stake. As I was not getting all the nutrients out of my food, I believe I basically had to eat more food to get the adequate nutrition.

Again, my work was suffering and I found I was not able to work very hard. I was very red in the face all the time and sweating profusely. I had very little zest for life and became frequently unemployed and unable to work.

I spoke to my doctor and he thought a change of PPI's might make a difference. I was eager to try. After only a few days on the new PPI's my face turned an even deeper shade of red. This was humiliating and very depressing. I threw the PPI's in the bin.

Chapter 10

H2 Blockers

Concerned that PPI's were killing me slowly, I changed over to a H2 blocker. I was able to buy these over the counter.

The color of my face returned to normal and this was a huge relief. Apart from my face I didn't notice much difference being on H2 blockers from PPI's but intuitively, I felt that the H2 blockers were better for me. I did notice that if I didn't take my H2 blocker on time, I definitely got a strong bout of heartburn.

Now in my mid 40's, I had a new health problem, anxiety. I think I knew already what was wrong. As I was approaching the same age as my half-brother was when he died, I was afraid that I too was going to die soon.

Over the years I had tried many different supplements for my health but I didn't notice any benefits. I started studying deficiencies and noticed that iodine and magnesium were very common deficiencies. I bought a kelp-supplement for iodine and I noticed improvements within a few weeks. My chronic back pain eased considerably and my elbow improved a little.

Then something wonderful happened. I had my nose broken very badly in a boxing match when I was twenty and I was never able to breathe through it properly since then. After a few weeks on the kelp-supplement I was able to breathe freely through my nose. This felt exhilarating but I wondered did it mean I was low in Iodine for 25 years?

The magnesium oil helped relax my muscles and contributed to a relaxing nights rest, coupled with the iodine, all this helped relieve my anxiety substantially.

It was really nice to experience a little good health after so many stressful years. On another positive note, my doctor had me on a list to have a gastroscopy and this was coming up soon.

Chapter 11

Centaurium

The nurse asked me if I wanted to forgo the anesthetic for the gastroscopy but my tears told her all she needed to know.

When I woke up, the specialist informed me that I had a hiatal hernia, so I knew now what was causing my heartburn. The only advice given to me was to stay on my medication and avoid smoking, so really, nothing changed.

One day as I was driving through the countryside, I popped into a health-shop to get my over-the-counter H2 blockers. The lady at the counter apologized for not having any left and offered an alternative medicine. I declined, explaining to her some of my previous experiences and I wanted to stick with the brand I was using.

We chatted a while and it was obvious to me that she knew a lot about heartburn. She explained to me that an older gentleman called in regularly to get a bottle of Centaurium for his heartburn, "Have you heard of it?". "No!", I exclaimed, genuinely surprised I hadn't heard of it after so many years of scanning the internet for information.

I asked her if she thought it would work on me as I had a hiatal hernia. She explained that the older gentleman also had the same condition. Whatever skepticism I had was overcome with enthusiasm and the lady ordered a bottle for me.

A few days later I picked up my bottle. Centaurium – Centaurium Umbellatum. When I stopped taking my H2 blockers I did get some very bad heartburn but within a couple of days the Centaurium did indeed work a treat. I cannot describe how happy I was to be able to change my medication for a natural remedy. The Centaurium drops tasted horrible but I put them into a glass of cola and had no problem consuming it. The little bottle lasted a long time so it worked out as inexpensive. If I missed a dose, I would definitely get heartburn so I bought a few bottles and always had one to hand.

My health improved very quickly. I was able to do a good hard day's work again and I felt strong for the first time in years.

Chapter 12

Comfrey

I believe my new found strength was as a direct result of digesting my food properly and getting the trace minerals and nutrients I was missing out on while on the H2 blockers and the PPI's.

During my many hours of surfing the internet for cures for the body, I had stumbled across a plant called comfrey. There is a long, long history of it being used to cure many ailments including stomach ailments so I decided I had to try this. It has been traditionally been called 'knitbone' so I assumed that it must have some power.

After many hours of studying comfrey and its uses on the internet, I bought two 500g bags of comfrey-root powder. Many articles explained to use it as a poultice, that is, externally applied. These same articles advised against using comfrey orally as it contains pyrrolizidine alkaloids that are potentially dangerous to the liver. However, the only way I read of consuming it orally was through comfrey tea which is made from the leaves and stems of the plant. Comfrey root is for external applications and you most certainly would not, or should not make tea from it.

Chapter 13

Application

My comfrey arrived but I really was not sure what to do with it. It is a dry powder. I poured some into a bowl with water and started mashing it up with a fork. It is not an easy substance to mix up into a paste suitable for an external application. If you try to mix it with a little water, it tends to 'cake-up' and becomes really difficult to mash.

After lots of trial and error I realized I was using too much comfrey in each mix and eventually learned that one full tablespoon was plenty for each application. I learned that a good dash of water to start with is much easier than trying to mash in a little water at a time. I bent a fork at the same angle as the side of the cereal-bowl I mixed it in and after a lot of practice I was able to mix up an application in a very short time.

Mixing up the comfrey-root powder was one thing, applying it was another. Most of the remedies I read about were poultices, wet rags holding the comfrey-root mixture to the target area.

It was not easy trying to place it in the middle of my chest just above the diaphragm. I was placing the application on wet rags on my lower chest but holding them there was difficult while I tried to put on a night shirt or pajama top. I then had to duct tape the outside of my pajama top to hold the rags in place. This did not work well. I was freezing cold at nights and the comfrey application was squeezing out and hardening on my pajamas.

A couple of times I placed the comfrey application on my chest and wrapped myself in cling-film. This held the comfrey application against my chest but it was uncomfortable.

After much trial and error, I eventually came up with a simpler system. I cut three strips of cling-film the full width or more of my chest. I overlapped two of them by six inches or so and then put the final strip in the middle to make a 'patch'. This was best done on a table to prevent the cling-film from 'gathering-up'. I placed the comfrey application in the middle of my cling-film patch, then, while leaning backwards slightly, placed the patch on my chest where the comfrey application was perfectly over the hiatal hernia. The cling-film, naturally clung to me, making it easier to put on a night-shirt. I was using old polo shirts at this stage because previously the comfrey application had escaped and hardened into my pajamas so by now, I was using the same old polo shirts each time.

Once I had my polo shirt on, I wrapped a full strip of duct-tape fully around my back and upper stomach just under the comfrey application. This generally stopped the comfrey application from leaking down.

Comfrey is an unusual substance, it tends to stay in one 'blob'. It is very hard to explain but when you use it a couple of times you will see it is a very workable substance.

Enough cling-film was showing through the 'v' in my polo shirt that I could put a strip of duct tape on it and the polo shirt, preventing the patch from slipping down.

Chapter 14

Cured

I had intended to apply the comfrey mixture every night but there were a lot of times I was too tired to go through the process and didn't want the hassle of cleaning up in the morning when I might have an earlier-than-usual start.

I used the comfrey-application about 4 or 5 nights a week. I put it on an hour or so before I went to bed. If I wasn't going anywhere in the morning, I tended to leave the application on till the afternoon.

After many weeks I noticed I needed less and less Centaurium drops to combat my heartburn. Then after 2 or 3 months or more, I noticed something very strange and worrying – The Centaurium drops were now *giving* me heartburn.

At a loss for what to do, I simply stopped taking the Centaurium. I braced myself for a terrible onslaught of heartburn but it never came. I spent some days living in worry, anticipating the heartburn before I remembered something I must have read somewhere. It was something along the lines of, 'After a medicine has cured you, that same medicine can now give you the symptoms you were initially using that medicine to treat'.

Quite simply, I was cured. I ceased applying the comfrey mixture and again I anticipated a terrible onslaught of heartburn but it never came. I was well and truly cured.

Chapter 15

Today

Today I am a healthy man. I still don't drink or smoke and I never will again. I still avoid all the 'triggers' even though I could probably eat and drink them now but I am too nervous to try them and I don't want to tempt fate. I did eat a full big-bag of crisps one day to see if it would give me heartburn, thankfully, it did not and that was the last time I ate crisps.

I have shed a lot of the excess weight I was carrying. I am able to fast now, something I could never do when I was suffering with heartburn. My mother noticed this about people with heartburn many years ago, they have to eat more often. If they fast for even a little while they get bad heartburn. I was eating over half of a loaf in toast every day when I used to suffer with heartburn. That is a lot of calories, especially when it was mostly marmalade I was using on the toast.

I have also given up tea and coffee. In hindsight I believe tea and coffee caused me quite a lot of heartburn. My stomach feels better without them. Notice I didn't say 'I have given up caffeine'. Both tea and coffee contain various different properties other than caffeine. The main reason I gave up tea and coffee was that I couldn't drink either without two spoons of sugar. At the rate I was drinking tea and coffee, I was consuming 20 teaspoons of sugar a day on top of everything else. Today I am happy not to be queuing up for coffee anywhere.

I drink sparkling water mixed with decaffeinated, diet coke now and I usually drink a glass of milk with meals.

I have practically given up all fruit and veg now and nobody is going to tell me that we need to be eating them at all. I get about one serving of veg a day and it is usually Brussels sprouts or cabbage because I like them and it easy to cook them one portion at a time.

Famed centenarian athlete Ruth Frith advised against eating vegetables and I am going to listen to someone who has lived as long and as healthily as her. Comedian James Gregory does a funny skit on 'fiber'. What makes most comedians work funny is that it is true.

I eat a Big Mac and three chicken selects at McDonald's almost every day, no fries. I look forward to this and I find it good value.

I still sleep in an inclined-bed, in fact I sleep in a reclining chair and I have never been more comfortable. I could never go back to sleeping in a regular bed.

A krill-oil supplement has helped my elbow further.

I am really happy to be alive and well today after those miserable years suffering with heartburn.

I hope that this book can cure others.

Made in United States
Orlando, FL
10 September 2024

51361341R00029